THE NEW FACE OF

DENTISTRY

A MULTIDISCIPLINARY APPROACH
TO WHOLE-BODY HEALTH

I0060715

LAURA TORRADO, DDS, FAGD

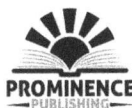

PROMINENCE
PUBLISHING

The New Face of Dentistry © Copyright 2025 by Dr. Laura Torrado

Published by Prominence Publishing.
Visit www.prominencepublishing.com.

The author can be reached as follows: info@drlauratorrado.com

The New Face of Dentistry/Dr. Laura Torrado. -- 1st ed.

ISBN: 978-1-990830-80-8

TABLE OF CONTENTS

Introduction

As a dentist with over three decades of experience, I have always been fascinated by the intricate connection between the face, jaws, and overall health. My journey began with a simple curiosity about the reasons behind the diverse facial structures I encountered as a child. I questioned what determined that our faces looked the way they look. What role did environment or genetics have in it? Sacred geometry and Chinese face reading were amusing and interesting topics. The DNA variants that offer so many different faces to look at fascinated me.

This curiosity led me to become a dentist. Then, it led me to explore beyond the conventional boundaries of dentistry and, ultimately, to discover a wholistic approach to treating patients. Addressing ostheopathic cranial patterns as they correlate to the rest of the body's health and well-being became the norm in my practice, but it is still not the norm in most dental settings.

Evaluating and treating the bite, cervical curvature, and body posture not only addresses dental problems related to TMD, recession, and airway incompetence but also correlates to the improvement of other general health issues. It was not our intention to practice outside the scope of dentistry, but the benefits came along and were welcomed by our patients.

In this book, I invite you to join me on a journey through the world of orthocranial dentistry. This approach focuses on understanding the underlying causes of dental issues and addressing them through a combination of cutting-edge technology, collaborative treatment, and a deep appreciation for the interconnectedness of the human body.

Through my 35 years of practice, I have witnessed first-hand the transformative power of orthocranial dentistry. Patients suffering from chronic pain, sleep disorders, and a host of other health issues have found relief and improved quality of life thanks to this wholistic approach.

In the following chapters, we will delve into the principles of this type of comprehensive dentistry, explore the importance of proper diagnosis, and discuss the practical applications of orthocranial treatment. We will also address common questions and concerns and showcase inspiring patient success stories.

As we embark on this journey together, I hope to shed light on this way of practicing dentistry and inspire a new generation of dentists and patients alike to embrace this transformative approach. Together, we can work toward a future where dental care is not just about fixing teeth but about promoting overall health and well-being.

"You can't have straight teeth on a crooked head!" I can hear my mentor telling me. "Look and diagnose the bigger picture."

CHAPTER 1

Understanding
Orthocranial Dentistry

In recent years, the field of dentistry has undergone a significant shift, moving away from a narrow focus on teeth and gums and towards a more comprehensive understanding of the intricate connections between mouth health and the rest of the body. At the forefront of this transformation is epigenetic and orthocranial dentistry—a science-based approach with a wholistic perspective of full body health and wellness from a cranial starting point.

We can trace the origins of orthocranial dentistry to Dr Sutherland, D.O. (1873–1954), an American osteopathic physician, and Andrew Taylor Still as the developers of all osteopathy, including the cranial approach. Sutherland described shape change in the bones of the cranium during breathing, and it was this motion that he called the body's "Primary Respiration." This is because the growth and development of the cranium into neutral or compensation patterns relates to the ability to exert proper respiration.

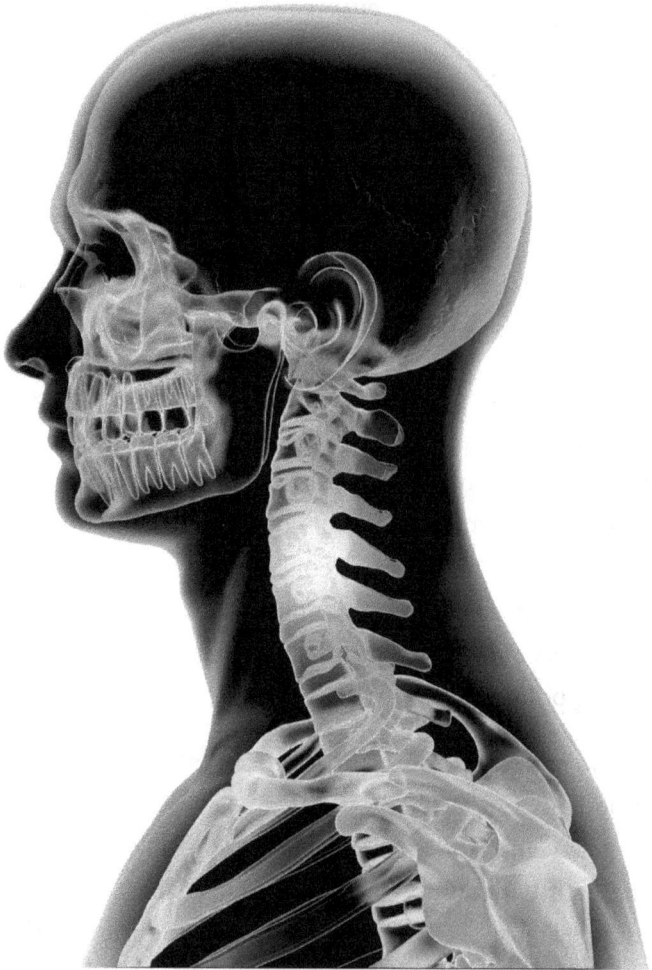

As dentists, we must take into account that the structure and function of the mouth, jaws, and cranial bones are deeply interconnected with overall health. Recognizing that dental problems such as malocclusion, temporomandibular joint disorders (TMD), and sleep apnea are not isolated issues but rather symptoms of underlying imbalances in the body is vital. Addressing these root causes of dental problems and alignment, rather than simply correcting the aesthetics of a bad bite, is at the core of true, comprehensive orthocranial dentistry.

Over the years, we have seen how conventional orthodontics, more often than not, address only teeth position and aesthetics without taking into account the future functionality of the entire stomatognatic system and as it relates to the rest of the body. Iatrogenesis is common in this field, leaving patients, through extraction-retraction orthodontics, with underdeveloped jaws and airways.

Children treated in this manner become sleep apnea and TMD patients, and reversing the damage done by stunting the growth of upper and lower jaws via extractions requires lengthy treatment of going back to braces and/or surgery. The use of CPAP/BIPAP machines to maintain proper oxygen levels is sometimes the only option as the interference with proper jaw development during childhood reduces the airway space and volume at the base of the tongue and the ability to inhale the proper volume of air needed for vital functioning is compromised. If there is intolerance to these devices (CPAP), the dentist will offer a nighttime mandibular advancement retainer to jut the lower jaw forward in order to open the airway passage to allow for better breathing. This device, in turn, could misalign the bite and have repercussions on the health of the temporomandibular joints, which could cause TMD and occlusion that will need to be treated at a later time.

As a profession, we know better now. This extraction-retraction modality is outdated, but many of our child patients are adults today who are suffering from problems stemming back to this surgical orthodontic modality during childhood treatment. Even so, I still get second-opinion consultations where some orthodontist has presented extractions as a viable option.

Considering factors such as facial development, airway function, and overall body posture is key for a successful treatment that supports overall health throughout a lifetime. Chronic pain, headaches, bad posture, sinus problems, sleep disorders, and even digestive issues are part of a cluster of signs and symptoms that arise from small jaws and airways. Patients who undergo orthocranial treatment often report significant improvements in their quality of life, with increased energy, better sleep, and a greater sense of overall well-being.

Maxillary morphogenesis, lower jaw repositioning, proper face height, TMD decompression, and occlusal restorative work are part of some of the comprehensive solutions that this modality offers to create more space for the tongue and teeth and to volumize the airway to optimize the function of the entire body through proper posture and efficient respiration. This wholistic approach recognizes the interconnectedness of the body and seeks to promote balance and harmony between the various systems.

In the following chapters, we will explore the principles and practices of orthocranial dentistry in greater detail, examining the science behind my approach and the practical applications for patients. As we delve deeper into the world of orthocranial dentistry, it becomes increasingly clear that this wholistic perspective represents the future of dental care—a future in which the mouth is seen not as an isolated entity but as a vital component of overall health and well-being.

CHAPTER 2

My Introduction to Orthocranial Dentistry

Many years ago, I was invited to audit a three-day weekend workshop on epigenetic dentistry in New York City. The workshop was organized by a company—still in existence today—that was promoting its own patented orthodontic dental device accessible to general dentists and orthodontists alike. Their goal was to improve patients' overall well-being, not just their jaws, by utilizing the concepts of applied epigenetic dentistry. The device had a catchy name, and I was curious to listen to the lectures and understand more about it.

The speakers presented a patented dental device designed with epigenetic principles in mind, which they claimed would promote bone remodeling in the mouth. They offered the opportunity for dentists to provide this device to their patients. However, I felt there wasn't enough assurance of proper training, and the proposal seemed overly focused on entrepreneurship rather than direct clinical patient care.

As I was leaving the lecture, I discussed the unusual financial approach of the company with another dentist also attending the lecture. We were concerned about the emphasis on corporate profiting from dentists implementing the use of the particular device rather than focusing on educating the dentist first in detail before utilizing it in direct patient care. It was then that he mentioned Dr. Theodore Belfor, saying, "He teaches the same concepts, but he is heavy on clinical knowledge and light on greed." This moment marked the beginning of my journey into the "New Face of Dentistry" approach to patient care.

I began to learn about dentofacial orthopedics, orthocranial dentistry, and the benefits of a properly aligned cervical spine, neutral cranial patterns, and a well-developed airway.

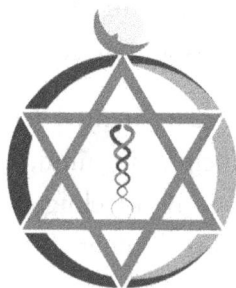

Dr. Ted Belfor opened a door to understanding true comprehensive dentistry within a multidisciplinary approach. His teachings also connected me to a talented and amazingly clinically knowledgeable postural restoration practitioner, Michal Niedzielski, PT. Through both Michal and Ted, I learned to look at patients wholistically, from head to toe and back up, even though I was primarily treating their mouths—or so I initially thought.

Today, we continue to deliver patient care that addresses both ascending and descending postural and cranial patterns—from cranium to feet and vice versa—with the goal of improving overall health and quality of life.

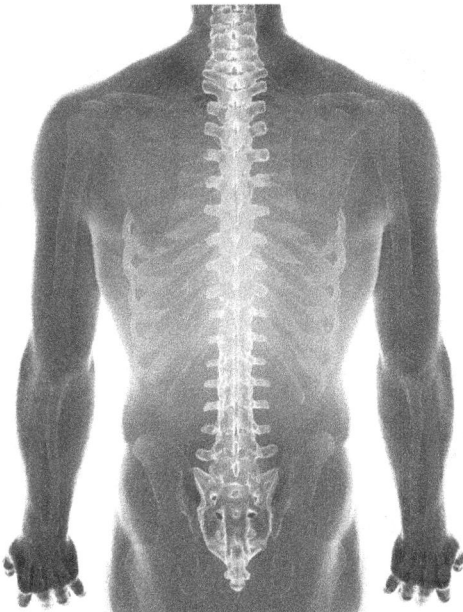

I began to study with Dr. Belfor, and it completely changed the trajectory of my career. I can still hear Dr. Ted telling me, "Laura, it's not only about teeth! Teeth just come along for the ride." As a dentist, I initially struggled with this concept. *What did he mean, "It's not about teeth?" I am a dentist Isn't that the sole focus of my profession?*

The key is to move beyond the old cookie-cutter modality of evaluating patients with the same dentally driven diagnostic tools. Instead, we need to start looking at the patient as a whole and knowing when to recruit complementary therapy modalities besides dentistry to achieve the desired goal of maximum medical and dental improvement.

Just as "cosmetic dentistry" boomed in the 80s and 90s, a new modality called "airway dentistry" has emerged. In 1991, the American Academy of Dental Sleep Medicine (AADSM) was established. Our patients want to breathe better despite generational trends towards smaller jaws and crowded teeth. The awareness of the importance of proper breathing and restorative sleep continues to expand, and consequently, the level of care that patients demand and receive continues to improve.

Books related to breathing techniques have proliferated, bringing awareness to the connection between jaws, breathing, and overall health. James Nestor's book,

Breath: New Science of a Lost Art (Riverhead 2020), and his personal experience with Dr. Belfor's treatment have brought immense awareness to the public. Patients now visit our practice from all over the world, curious about how they can improve their breathing, alleviate both TMD and cervical pain, correct their posture, and optimize their overall health.

People want to breathe! Who knew?

Meanwhile, dental devices promoted on social media to "define the angle of the lower jaw and cheek contouring" target the public interested mainly in aesthetics rather than function. Unfortunately, the potential overloading of the temporomandibular joint (TMJ) with consequent damage doesn't seem to matter to some as long as a chiseled jaw provides improved aesthetics. Requests to "order and deliver" this type of device with the idea that one design and size fits all are common in our practice, leaving us to explain that detailed diagnostics and custom measurements and fabrication of such devices are the only route to obtain any dental/medical grade appliance.

CHAPTER 3

How is the New Face of Dentistry Shaping Dental Visits and Overall Health?

An accurate diagnosis is crucial in determining the best treatment protocol for each patient. We consider what we need to achieve and which treatment options are most suitable for the specific patient. We then utilize the most adequate device and implement the proper technique needed to get the ideal result for each individual. "Patients are not born with an acrylic or metal deficiency," says one of my teachers.

We have only one most important goal from one minute to the next, and that is to be able to breathe. A survival instinct will make our bodies adapt and compensate in different ways. The consequences of that adaptation will manifest in different cranial patterns, bad posture, and a nervous system that stays in sympathetic/fight or flight mode with no hope of recovery, burning the candle through both ends.

So, where and how do we start in the treatment of these patients? A thorough evaluation is necessary, and technology and critical thinking must be applied to each case. We typically divide the treatment into two stages:

STAGE I

This stage focuses on bringing upper and lower jaws into alignment through maxillary morphogenesis and joint healing. This process is aided by full-body postural restoration therapy and even occasionally proper visual inputs with the help of a behavioral optometrist.

STAGE II

In this stage, when Maximum Medical Improvement (MMI) is achieved for the jaws and posture, a discussion of proper teeth alignment and restorative dentistry follows. Deciding when it is the appropriate time to proceed to Stage II is key. There are cases that require surgery on Stage I before we get here, and that will be presented at the diagnostic and discussion appointment.

The need for retainers is rare if we can maximize cranial and body neutrality, allowing the body to function with minimal compensation. By altering the proportions of the face to increase symmetry and repositioning the lower and upper jaws tri dimensionally we reduce the compensatory patterns that the body has to develop to function. These patterns overload the nervous and muscular system creating taxing demands on the body. Alignment and neutrality is the optimal functional goal. Neutrality aids in creating a more patent oropharyngeal space that allows more air volume at the base of the tongue and consequently into our lungs, causing the oropharyngeal space to expand laterally and creating a patent airway at the base of the tongue.

CHAPTER 4

WHY and HOW We Do What We Do

The continuous practice of conventional restorative dentistry seemed limiting to me as it did not address why teeth were wearing off unevenly or breaking, nor did it offer insights into a more wholistic patient care approach. Orthocranial dentistry transformed our practice rapidly, and today, we are providing comprehensive dental care in innovative ways with excellent results for our patients.

WHY

We practice this approach because it addresses complex dental problems at the root of cranial and postural issues, not just at the root of the tooth. Being an outlier in providing dental care while getting results that exceed patients' expectations is forever rewarding. I am continually grateful for being guided into this path.

HOW

1. **Detailed intake forms:** This is the first essential step, letting us know why patients are here and what they expect from us.

2. **Accurate diagnosis:** You only see what you know, and once seen, it can't be unseen.

3. **Treatment planning:** This is honed by accurate data collection and its analysis, plus carefully listening to our patients' consultation reasons and expectations of the actual treatment.

Technology plays a crucial role in our diagnostic process. Using a CBCT scanner has been essential to our office. The cone beam CT (Computer Aided Tomography or "CAT Scan") allows for the three-dimensional evaluation of the hard and certain soft tissues of the head and neck area. Each cone beam CT allows for the evaluation of the following structures:

- Temporomandibular joints for arthritis changes and joint position

- Para-nasal sinuses for chronic or acute sinus problems/infection

- Nasal septum for deviation

- Teeth and periodontal tissues for cavities, abscesses, bone loss, etc.

- Tongue for its position and airway for possible obstruction

- Cervical spine to approximately the 3rd or 4th vertebrae for arthritis changes and possible nerve impingement

- Facial bones and jaw bones for any fractures or lesions

- Bones and hard tissues of the ear for any abnormalities

- Styloid process for elongation or evidence of fracture

- Carotid artery blockages or stenosis

The cone beam CT allows for all of these structures to be evaluated with a single scan, providing very fine detail and allowing for measurements to be taken. It also involves very minimal radiation exposure for the patient. Each scan is utilized for a comprehensive evaluation, and all findings are discussed with the patient in detail at a separate appointment. A radiologist also reads the scan and certifies pre-treatment findings.

ADDITIONAL DIAGNOSTIC TOOLS INCLUDE:

- Digital scanning of all dental structures (teeth and gums)

- Intra and extraoral photography

- Analog records taken with models mounted on an articulator

- Analyze® software for advanced biomedical imaging visualization, manipulation, and measurement

- Exocad and 3Shape design software for the creation of our dental devices

- Bite registrations to understand jaw relationships

- Bite Analysis with T Scan software

These comprehensive diagnostic techniques allow us to provide a thorough and personalized approach to each patient's dental health and overall well-being.

FABRICATION OF THE APPLIANCES

We have incorporated 3D printing in our office. The accuracy of the design via different software packages has made the delivery of our dental devices more efficient.

As technology keeps advancing and we keep embracing it, the benefit for the patient is clear. Storing digital files allows for easier comparative models from beginning to end and seamless evaluation of before and after treatment results.

LET'S TALK ABOUT THE SPHENOID BONE: THE MOTHERBOARD OF THE CRANIUM

Sphenoid Bone Anatomy
(Anterior View)

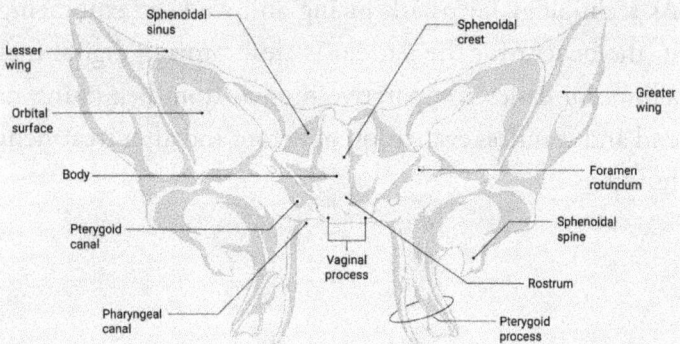

In the middle of the cranium lies the commander of our cranial system: the sphenoid bone. The sphenoid bone is my favorite skull bone. It serves as the motherboard connecting physicality to consciousness by holding space in the sella turcica for the pituitary gland, the master gland for hormonal production in the entire body. When the sphenoid is out of alignment, it's easy to see how the proper function of all nerves, arteries, and veins passing through it could be affected.

This remarkable structure serves as a crucial hub for a bundle of cranial nerves that pass through it. These include the:

- optic nerve (CN II)
- oculomotor nerve (CN III)
- trochlear nerve (CN IV)
- ophthalmic nerve (CN V1)
- abducens nerve (CN VI)
- sympathetic fibers from the cavernous plexus

Additionally, the maxillary division of the trigeminal nerve (CN V2), the mandibular division of the trigeminal nerve (CN V3), the motor root of the trigeminal nerve, and the lesser petrosal nerve pass through this region, along with the meningeal branch of the mandibular nerve.

The sphenoid bone, shaped like a butterfly, bears a striking resemblance to many structures in nature that hold sacred geometry arrangements. From its central position, it commands and influences exquisite bodily functions. Given its critical role, it's logical to consider that a sphenoid bone out of alignment could have significant repercussions on our overall cranial health and full-body well-being.

When the sphenoid is out of neutral position, it can deviate the passage of the ocular nerve. This misalignment impacts how we perceive ourselves in space and how we perceive our surroundings, ultimately affecting our posture and gait. Furthermore, a tilted maxillary upper arch will determine the traveling path that the lower jaw must follow to meet the upper teeth, essentially finding the top of the head.

If the mandible follows a wavy path upward instead of a centered and aligned one, it will pull on the neck muscles in an unbalanced manner. This imbalance affects the cervical spine and temporomandibular joints. The jaw's posture has far-reaching effects, influencing the shoulder grid, hips, and foot stance. Consequently, the bite determines how your feet land on the ground via the shoulder grid and hips, while your feet, in turn, influence your hip, spinal column, neck, and jaw posture in relation to your cranium.

Deciding where to start treatment requires careful analysis. We must determine whether it's an ascending pattern that needs correction (from feet up to cranium) or a descending pattern (where the misaligned cranium determines the posture of the body as a whole).

In a well designed structural architectural plan, bones should be in postural neutrality so they allow, muscles and the vessels and nerves that traverse through without compensation. This neutral state allows the body to operate in high-efficiency mode. It's worth noting that athletes with high-performance abilities typically have the least compensatory patterns of posture and breathing, illustrating the importance of proper alignment.

Five Neuromuscular Structural Planes

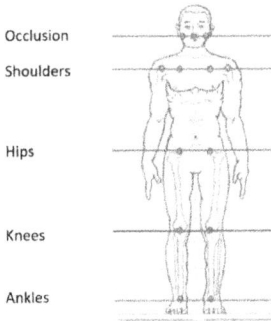

CHAPTER 5

So, Where Do We Start?

As dentists, we begin from the top, focusing on the cranium and jaws. Proper referrals will follow to achieve full body optimization. During the initial dental evaluation, if signs and symptoms suggest the need for physical therapy due to evident body misalignment or pain, both dental and physical therapy treatments may be implemented simultaneously.

The dentist and the physical therapist will have joint sessions with the patient. As the body receives alignment via physical therapies and curated exercises, the dental alignment devices will need to be properly adjusted. Body posture changes will then affect mandibular and maxillary alignment.

In our current healthcare system, where corporate profits often prevail over patient health benefits, preventive medicine protocols are not always prioritized. For example, amputating a leg may be more profitable than teaching the importance of early detection of insulin resistance. This profit-driven approach often results in a lack of seamless cross-referrals between healthcare providers.

Communication gaps are common, even between specialties within dentistry. Minimizing this hurdle is at the core of our protocol. Working collaboratively with physical therapists, ENTs, craniosacral therapists, acupuncturists, and other specialists is key to overall success. Patients must be their own health advocates, and spending adequate time educating them is crucial to obtaining the best results.

"Position gives you power," says Michal. Determining the alignment of the 22 bones in your skull through 3D imaging and its analysis is the starting point of our evaluation. Ideally, the ocular, otic, and occlusal planes should be parallel to each other and to the floor. We assess whether their alignment allows for proper functioning in synchronicity with the surrounding structures and if they are functioning in opposition to or in tandem with each other.

We recruit concepts from aeronautics to define the performance and alignment of the cranium: pitch, roll, and yaw. Osteopathy measures these aspects to determine how far from center and neutrality the structures around and inside the cranium are functioning or compensating and how much torque the dura of the brain is subjected to with repercussions on neural functioning.

The design of the treatment plan will take into consideration the extent of deviation from the ideal and the realistic Maximum Medical Improvement (MMI) possible.

ANALYSIS AND EVALUATION FROM THE TOP DOWN

Initial data collection, as described earlier, helps us determine the shape and position of the entire cranium. To use a common language, we employ the classification of osteopathic cranial patterns: left and right side bending, torsion, and inferior and superior vertical strain. Deviations from the norm or ideal are noted.

We assess:

- ✓ The location of the joints

- ✓ The bite, neck, and tongue position

- ✓ Define cranial patterns and compensatory patterns

- ✓ Radiological analysis by referral to a certified radiologist

- ✓ Nasal passages and sinus health

✓ Cephalometrics to evaluate deviation from ideal

✓ 3D printed models of both jaws and bite registration to articulate and visualize upper and lower jaw positions in 3D space

Each compensatory pattern provides a script for the healing path to follow, guiding us on how to bring the 22 bones in your cranium into the best possible alignment as they relate to your cervical spine and the rest of the body and the occlusal/bite scheme.

WHY IS TONGUE POSTURE SO IMPORTANT?

The human tongue, as a hydrostatic diaphragm, provides skeletal support for motion through muscle contraction. It doesn't develop around any particular bone, and the architecture of its muscle fibers forms the basis for hydrostatic deformation. Toning the base of the tongue with myofunctional and appliance therapy directly affects the size and patency of airway passages, promoting efficient breathing.

The tongue's attachment to the inside of the jaw also has a direct connection through fascia to the thoracic and pelvic regions. This means that restricted tongue movement can affect breathing and pelvic health. Therefore, the evaluation of tongue-tie and restricted tongue movement is part of our comprehensive assessment.

Open bites in babies and improper tongue posture can lead to immature swallowing and improper lip and oropharyngeal seals. This is important because the quality of body and tongue posture directly affects the quality of life, potentially causing a shift from a parasympathetic response of balance, rest, and digestion to a sympathetic "fight or flight" response. This causes increased cortisol levels, which leads to increased heart and respiratory rates and higher stress levels.

Early extraction retraction orthodontics in children can cause permanent damage, potentially turning ortho-dontic patients into sleep apnea patients by stunting the proper growth of upper and lower jaws.

DOES MY INSURANCE COVER IT?

Dental insurance coverage is limited, and many policies don't include adult orthodontic and TMD treatment, which are the categories under which these services would typically be billed. If dental insurance had kept pace with the cost of living since its inception in the 1950s, each patient should have no less than $25,000 in yearly benefits today. Unfortunately, such comprehensive coverage is nonexistent.

The dental code for orthodontics in adults is D8090, and for TMD, the code is D7880 Occlusal Orthotic Device. You can ask your insurance what type of coverage you have for those to get a clear understanding of where you stand.

HOW DOES IT LOOK?

The initial treatment typically involves a dental device for the upper jaw that can be used at night and a full arch splint for the lower jaw during the day. The nighttime device aids in maxillary morphogenesis by rounding the upper arch with a more viable U shape that is more conducive to proper tongue posture. The visibility of these appliances during speech and smiling varies depending on the patient.

A WORD ON THE PINEAL GLAND

STIMULATION AND CALCIFICATION:

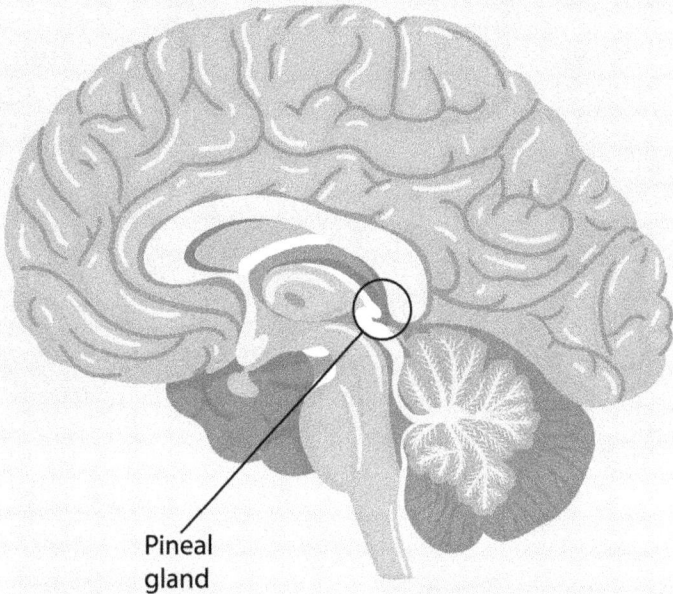

Pineal
gland

While the exact function of the pineal gland remains unclear, it's often considered a mystical bridge between physical and spiritual consciousness, with piezoelectric properties. We can postulate that compensatory cranial patterns out of neutral, generating mechanical stress, could have a direct effect on pineal gland function.

CHAPTER 6

The New Face of Dentistry: Epigenetic Approach

Epigenetic dentistry represents a paradigm shift in the way we think about oral health and its connection to overall well-being. By focusing on the intricate relationships between the teeth, jaws, and surrounding structures, this approach offers a more comprehensive understanding of the causes of dental problems and guides the treatment.

At the core of our approach is the recognition that the mouth is not an isolated entity but rather an integral part of a complex and interconnected system. The position and function of the teeth and jaws are deeply influenced by the alignment of the cranial bones, the posture of the body, and the function of the airway and surrounding muscles.

One of the key principles of epigenetic dentistry is the idea that malocclusion, or misalignment of the teeth, is not simply an aesthetic issue but rather a symptom of underlying imbalances in the craniofacial complex. As mentioned, when the jaws are underdeveloped or misaligned, it can lead to a host of secondary problems, from TMD and headaches to sleep apnea and postural issues.

By addressing these underlying imbalances through a combination of specialized appliances, functional exercises, and other targeted interventions, dentists aim to promote proper facial development and restructuring that supports optimal health and wellness.

One of the most important aspects of our approach is the emphasis on collaboration with other healthcare providers. Because the mouth and jaws are so intimately connected with the rest of the body, effective treatment often requires a multidisciplinary approach that involves input from a range of specialists, like postural restoration doctors, to address imbalances in body posture and alignment. We also collaborate with ENTs (ear, nose, and throat specialists) to evaluate and treat issues related to the airway and breathing, such as sleep apnea and chronic sinusitis.

We also work closely with craniosacral therapists, who specialize in promoting balance and harmony in the cranial bones and surrounding tissues. By addressing restrictions and imbalances in the craniosacral system, these therapists can support the body's natural healing processes and promote optimal function. Redesigning the shape of both upper and lower dental arches and promoting proper tongue posture; treatment can help improve breathing and reduce the risk of sleep apnea. By correcting jaw misalignment in this way and promoting proper bite function, we can alleviate TMD symptoms and reduce the risk of chronic pain and headaches.

As the field of dentistry continues to evolve, we hope that this comprehensive approach becomes the standard of care rather than a unique protocol implemented by a few dentists.

BEFORE YOU START A YOGA PRACTICE, DO YOU KNOW YOUR CRANIAL PATTERN AND COMPENSATORY BODY PATTERN?

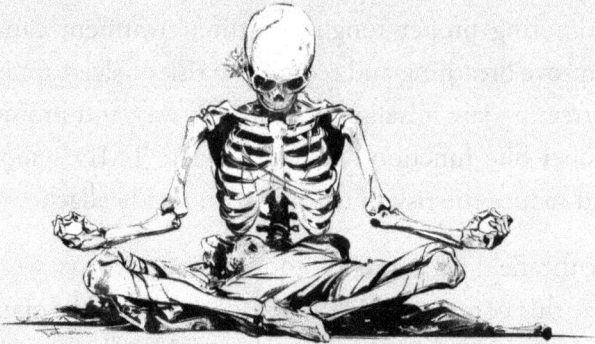

The asanas in yoga were created by male yogis in Northern India around 2,700 BC to withstand hours of meditation in stillness. Their jaws did not have crowded teeth, unlike modern populations affected by dietary changes, improper breathing, and swallowing habits brought on by the agricultural and industrial revolutions and overconsumption of sugar.

Forward head posture to compensate for a diminished airway size is a common adaptation and can be difficult to overcome when attempting certain yoga positions.

Asanas that demand a "no pain, no gain" approach might be more damaging than beneficial if we're not aware of existing pathocompensatory cranial patterns. Each cranial pattern will have repercussions on body posture. Some yoga practices disregard these adaptations of the body, and they might create more damage than benefit.

CHAPTER 7

Treatment Protocols and Techniques

Orthocranial dentistry employs a range of specialized treatment protocols and techniques designed to promote optimal facial development and function.

One of the key tools used in orthocranial dentistry is the Homeoblock appliance, developed by Dr. Theodore Belfor. This custom-made, removable device is designed to promote proper jaw remodeling, cranial pattern correction, and alignment by gently stimulating the mesenchymal cells within the periodontal ligament of the teeth. By encouraging the remodeling of new bone and reshaping the dental arches, the Homeoblock can help correct malocclusion, improve breathing and sleep quality, and alleviate dysautonomia.

Another important appliance used in epigenetic dentistry is the Bioblock, which is similar in design to the Homeoblock with a midpalatal screw and front wires that get activated with proper swallow. An ALF (advanced lightwire functional) and three-way sagittal devices are also part of the arsenal of devices that we can use to implement treatment.

Throughout the treatment process of bone remodeling and displacement, the orthocranial dentist works closely with their patients to monitor the progress of palatal remodeling, TMD healing, lower jaw repositioning, and tooth movement. Adjustments will be needed as treatment progresses and when postural restoration exercises are implemented. The length of treatment can vary depending on the individual patient's needs and goals but typically ranges from 18 to 24 months.

While orthocranial dentistry offers a range of promising benefits, it is important to recognize that, like any medical intervention, it also has its limitations and potential challenges. The success of treatment may depend on factors such as patient compliance, overall health status, and the severity of the underlying dental problems. Not all patients might be candidates for the treatment.

Not all dentists are trained in these techniques, and access to care may be limited in some areas. We have patients from all over the world coming to our clinic in Manhattan. As with any healthcare decision, it is important for patients to carefully consider their options, discuss the potential risks and benefits with their provider, and make an informed choice based on their individual needs and circumstances. Despite these challenges, orthocranial dentistry significantly improves overall well-being and function, starting at the cranium.

CHAPTER 8

Frequently Asked Questions

Patients considering orthocranial dentistry often have a range of questions and concerns. In this chapter, we will address some of the most common queries and misconceptions about this approach in order to provide a clear and comprehensive understanding of this exciting field.

1. *Can I show this to my dentist? My father is a dentist. I need a copy of the scan and evaluation.*

    Yes, you can show this to your dentist. However, it's important to consider what kind of training in orthocranial dentistry they have that would allow for a valid second opinion. Does your dentist know about cranial osteopathy and how different cranial patterns affect the bite, TMJ, cervical spine, general posture, and the rest of the body?

2. *What is orthocranial dentistry?*

Orthocranial dentistry takes into account craniometrics and body posture for diagnosis before attempting to create a treatment plan. In traditional dental education, we are trained to limit our view to teeth and jaws as if they are not related to the rest of the skull and body. Orthocranial dentistry offers a more comprehensive approach, moving away from the very segmented and mechanistic view of the body typically taught in dental schools. Tapping into epigenetics, the concept of the body healing the body when given more ideal conditions, becomes second nature in this approach.

3. *What courses have you taken, and what education is out there to become an orthocranial dentist?*

I have taken courses with the American Academy of Craniofacial Pain (AACFP), completed sleep medicine and TMD courses at Tufts University, and received training from Dr. Ted Belfor, Dr. Bob Walker, and Michal Niedzielski. I am a graduate of the Kois Institute in Seattle, a Fellow of the Academy of General Dentistry, and a Pankey Institute scholar.

4. Are you sure I can grow bone?

The proper term is maxillary morphogenesis. This process involves the displacement of the entire alveolus (the bone casing that holds the entire tooth) in a lateral fashion. This allows for a wider roof of the mouth, which in turn provides more space for the tongue to rest in a better position: forward and out of the airway. This positioning allows for the proper function of the tongue as a hydrostatic diaphragm and a mature swallow.

5. Would I be able to get rid of the CPAP that I use for my sleep apnea?

While I can't make definitive claims, many patients obtain improvement in airway size and volumetric capacity through repositioning of the lower jaw and widening of the roof of the mouth. This can facilitate down-titration of the CPAP to a lesser amount of airflow needed. In many instances, snoring is eliminated.

6. I am desperate. I need to stop the pain. I have tried everything with little results. Will this work for me?

A proper diagnosis will determine if you are a candidate for this treatment. Sometimes, the ultimate solution is orthognathic surgery with pre-surgery functional treatment indicated. This may include maximum maxillary morphogenesis, lower jaw repositioning, postural restoration, and fixed orthodontics.

7. How often do I need to see you?

After delivery of the dental appliances and a fit check, your next appointment will be 30 days later to ensure they are being used properly. Within 2-3 months of using the devices, we recommend a visit with the postural restoration/PT provider in our office. This visit will determine the ideal schedule for you to see us in person. At 12 months, a new scan and reevaluation are needed to check progress and determine if we need to incorporate further treatment modalities or if what's being done is sufficient, having achieved the maximum improvement possible.

8. Why aren't all dentists doing this?

This approach requires specialized, detailed post-graduate training that is not easily found. The limited availability of courses and exposure to the subject in continued dental education circles might be a determinant as to why there are not many dentists practicing in this manner.

9. *How do I know that this is for me?*

The evaluation, discussion of findings, and proposed treatment will yield all the answers you need to determine if this approach is right for you.

10. *What symptoms have you seen most improved or eradicated?*

We've observed improvements in full body posture, tongue posture, breathing, TMD symptoms, sleep efficiency, and pain reduction or elimination. Patients start to feel better, and it shows in their demeanor and outlook. Living with pain and suboptimal breathing is debilitating. We've also seen diminished central nervous system sensitization with all associated symptoms, as well as improvement or elimination of IBS and other digestive issues.

11. *Does the treatment hurt?*

No, the treatment doesn't hurt. We use very low cyclical forces created by the tongue during swallowing to stimulate the mesenchymal cells in the periodontal ligament to stimulate bone remodeling. The daytime splint aids in lower jaw position and full body posture as well as TMJ condylar remodeling.

12. *How far into treatment could I expect to start experiencing relief from symptoms?*

We expect noticeable improvement within a few weeks of starting the therapy if the patient is following the protocol. In instances where this is not the case, it's most often due to a lack of compliance. At three to four months, the difference should be noticeable.

13. *My chief concerns are clicking, popping, and pressure in my ears; snoring and waking up feeling unrested; difficulty falling asleep; receding and sensitive bleeding gums; headaches; and jaw pain. Can I expect the treatment plan will address these symptoms?*

Yes, these are exactly some of the symptoms that our treatment addresses. All of these concerns will be discussed during the initial evaluation, diagnosis, and presentation of the treatment plan.

14. *I was given a mouth guard a while back, and it caused me to have even more headaches and jaw pain. Is there a possibility that the appliance you're prescribing could have that same effect? If so, what would be the remedy?*

Without seeing what type of appliance you received, it's hard to determine the cause of the adverse effects, as well as the conditions of your body at that time. The appliance and treatment plan we recommend is designed to improve the conditions you've stated, not to produce harm or adverse effects. It's rare for our treatment to cause such issues, as it's a pretty straightforward choice of treatment once we get the proper diagnosis.

15. How long do I have to be under treatment?

In general, the treatment lasts 18 to 24 months.

16. After we are done, do I use a retainer?

A removable nighttime guard is recommended but not mandatory. If the body has been brought into alignment, there's no need to "retain." Optimization and better posture are maintained without the need for extra forces.

17. Why do I need to see a postural restoration doctor? I just came to the dentist.

The cranium is connected to the rest of the body, and the position of the jaw and head will determine the position of your shoulder grid, hips, and feet. In a descending pattern, how your teeth meet affects how you stand in relation to the floor and vice versa. We call these descending patterns (cranium down) or ascending patterns (feet up). We are one unit, not segmented parts trying to work together. Each body part knows what the other is doing.

18. I am upset that I just came to the dentist and now have to spend money on a PT, a behavioral optometrist, and shoe inserts! Someone has to take ownership of this!

Yes, the patient has to take ownership of their problems and have the gratitude and willingness to work towards a healthier body and mind. The treatment is optional, not compulsory. A comprehensive multidisciplinary treatment is better than a reductionist approach. You are being treated as a whole person, not just a set of teeth.

19. How much does it cost?

Proper care, skill, and clinical judgment are not acquired overnight. Delivery of such by a healthcare provider is reflected in the fees. Faster and cheaper has never been good. Fortunately, payment plans are available.

20. How come we get results without regular braces? Is it true?

We address bone alignment and posture first, then the teeth will follow. Clear braces for a short amount of time are sometimes needed at the end.

21. *Is there an online community for support where I can ask for feedback from others who are experiencing the treatment?*

An online community for support is currently under development.

22. *This is a two-year commitment? I hope you are not retiring soon.*

We will make sure that your treatment is successfully completed under proper supervision. There are no plans for retirement at the moment.

23. *How would I look while I am using the appliances? I do a lot of talking for work. I need to be able to function.*

There will be a period where you will be "under construction." The appliances are removable if there is an absolute need to take them off. A slight delay in treatment will occur if there are continuous gaps in usage, but they don't interfere with regular life. This is temporary.

24. *Do you use a local lab? Who makes these devices?*

The devices are made right in New York City, where our offices are located. Some devices are 3D printed in-office.

25. Are there patents for these devices, and who owns them?

The Homeoblock was initially patented by Dr. Belfor more than 20 years ago. Other devices we use, like the Bioblock, Schwartz appliances, and occlusal splints, have been tools in the world of dentistry for years.

26. What is your background, and how did you come to do this type of dentistry?

I am a foreign graduate dentist from Uruguay and completed my U.S. education at NYU College of Dentistry. After 30 years of practicing general dentistry in the United States, I was introduced to the field of orthocranial dentistry by Dr. Belfor and Michal Niedzielski. This knowledge allows me to connect the dots between dental and full-body optimization and function. Cooperation with other non-dental providers is key. Starting from a cranio-dental diagnosis, we now treat patients comprehensively, connecting dental health with full-body well-being.

27. Do the profession and dental boards support this integrative way of practicing?

This approach is indeed within the scope of dentistry, and collaboration with other healthcare providers completes the circle of care. Conventional orthodontics mostly addresses tooth positioning without regard to cranial patterns. You can't have straight teeth on a crooked head, and diagnosis of cranial patterns, jaw posture, swallowing patterns, and breathing patterns is a must for successful treatment.

28. How does the advent of corporate dentistry affect this approach?

The demand for faster and cheaper treatments, plus limited insurance coverage in general, challenges the widespread implementation of this modality. The lack of public education about the connection between crooked teeth, jaw positioning, developmental issues, and breathing should be improved to ensure this method is more widely implemented.

29. How do you ensure patients understand their conditions and treatment options?

The patient isn't ready to heal until they understand their conditions and what can be done to make them better. Co-discovery during examinations utilizing extensive collected data has been key in raising awareness. Many patients are surprised to discover the reasons for their upper airway resistance. They have lived all their lives with suboptimal function and have assumed that it was the only way.

Ownership and understanding of their diagnosis lays the foundation for patient cooperation in their treatment. All questions are answered, all options are presented, and all expected outcomes are discussed.

CHAPTER 9

Patient Success Stories

One of the most compelling aspects of orthocranial dentistry is the profound impact it can have on patients' lives. By addressing the underlying causes of dental problems and promoting optimal health and wellness, orthocranial treatment has helped countless individuals overcome chronic pain, improve their breathing and sleep quality, and enhance their overall quality of life.

In this chapter, we will share some inspiring stories from patients who have experienced firsthand the transformative power of orthocranial dentistry. These stories offer a glimpse into the wide range of benefits that orthocranial treatment can provide and highlight the importance of a wholistic, patient-centered approach to dental care. All the names in the following stories have been changed to ensure patient privacy, but each one is a very real example of the life-altering improvement patients have experienced after treatment.

SARAH WITH SLEEP APNEA

Sarah had been struggling with sleep apnea for years. Every night, she'd strap on her CPAP machine, feeling like a scuba diver in her own bed. After researching alternative treatments, she decided to try maxillary morphogenesis.

For a year, Sarah diligently used the Homeoblock device, which gradually widened her palate. The process wasn't always comfortable, but Sarah persevered, hoping for a breakthrough. A jaw repositioning splint and full-body postural restoration therapy were implemented.

Finally, after 15 months, and with improved tongue posture, she underwent another sleep study. To her amazement and delight, the results showed that her apneic events had been reduced to zero.

For the first time in years, Sarah experienced truly restful sleep without the need for her CPAP machine. A copy of her report without her name is included on page 68.

MARIEL WITH NECK PAIN

Mariel had always been self-conscious about her smile. As a teenager, she underwent extraction retraction orthodontics, a common practice at the time. While her teeth looked straighter, she began experiencing persistent neck pain in her early twenties.

Unbeknownst to Mariel, the orthodontic procedure had stunted the growth of her upper and lower jaws, reducing the size of her airway. Her body, desperately seeking oxygen, compensated by developing a forward head posture. This postural change allowed her to breathe more easily, but it came at the cost of chronic neck pain and tension headaches.

It wasn't until Mariel sought help from an orthocranial dentist that she understood the root cause of her discomfort and began a journey to correct the unintended consequences of her childhood orthodontic treatment.

NICO WAS IMBALANCED

Nico was a dedicated triathlete, always pushing himself to improve his performance. However, despite his rigorous training regimen, he felt like he had hit a plateau. What Nico didn't realize was that the extraction orthodontics he had undergone as a child had created subtle but significant imbalances in his body.

Seeking to gain an edge in his competitions, Nico began working with Michal on postural restoration while simultaneously undergoing treatment to remodel his jaw position and posture. The team also brought in a behavioral optometrist who prescribed special glasses to provide Nico's brain with better information about his surroundings.

The results were remarkable. In his next competition, Nico shaved minutes off his previous best time. As he continued with the treatment, he found himself consistently performing better in all aspects of his triathlons—swimming, cycling, and running. Nico's story became a testament to the far-reaching effects of proper jaw alignment and posture on athletic performance.

CELESTE WITH SCOLIOSIS

Celeste had lived with scoliosis for most of her life, enduring chronic pain and limited mobility. When she first heard about maxillary morphogenesis and jaw repositioning as a potential aid for her condition, she was skeptical but willing to try anything for relief.

The treatment began with widening her palate, followed by carefully repositioning her jaw. This allowed for TMJ decompression and remodeling, which in turn facilitated the regaining of a healthier cervical curvature. As the weeks turned into months, Celeste noticed gradual improvements. Her posture began to straighten, and the constant ache in her back started to diminish.

While the treatment wasn't a cure for her scoliosis, it provided Celeste with significant pain relief and improved her quality of life in ways she hadn't thought possible.

ASHELY HAD BREATHING DIFFICULTIES

Ashley, a personal trainer, prides herself on her physical fitness and body awareness. However, she had always struggled with certain exercises and couldn't understand why. After undergoing a comprehensive cranial assessment, it was discovered that her cranial pattern was contributing to poor posture and inefficient breathing.

Ashley embarked on a treatment plan that included palatal expansion and jaw repositioning. As her treatment progressed, she noticed remarkable changes in her body. Her posture improved naturally, without conscious effort, and she found herself breathing more deeply and efficiently during workouts. These changes translated into improved performance in her training sessions and a newfound ability to demonstrate and perform exercises that had previously been challenging.

Ashley's experience not only improved her personal fitness but also made her a more effective trainer for her clients.

SILVIA WITH EHLERS-DANLOS SYNDROME

Sylvia, a dedicated yoga teacher, faced unique challenges due to her Ehlers-Danlos syndrome (EDS), a condition affecting connective tissue. EDS causes faster movements in tooth positioning and shaping the dental arches.

However, achieving maximum medical improvement (MMI) proved difficult due to her condition's effect on her overall body posture.

It wasn't until a coordinated approach was implemented, combining cranial manipulation with specialized postural restoration exercises tailored to her Ehlers-Danlos syndrome and adding height to her bite, that Silvia began to see significant improvements.

This experience not only enhanced Silvia's personal practice but also deepened her understanding of the body's interconnectedness, enriching her teaching and allowing her to better assist students with similar challenges.

SUZANNE AND CHRISTINE HAD CHRONIC HEADACHES

The stories of Suzanne and Christine further illustrate the immediate impact of proper jaw positioning. Both women had suffered from chronic jaw pain and tension headaches for years. When they were fitted with dental devices designed to allow for proper jaw posture and maxillary morphogenesis, the relief was almost instantaneous.

Suzanne described it as "like a weight being lifted off my face," while Christine noted that for the first time in years, she could open her mouth wide without wincing.

Their experiences highlight the profound effect that seemingly small adjustments can have on overall comfort and well-being.

* * * *

These cases collectively demonstrate a crucial principle: What happens in the cranium and cervical spine has far-reaching repercussions throughout the body. From top to bottom, and vice versa, kinetic muscle chains connect various body parts. When one part of the chain functions more efficiently, it positively impacts the entire system, creating a sense of coherence and balance in the body.

While jaw repositioning and cranial alignment are just one piece of the puzzle in optimizing bodily function, these stories show how this piece can be a critical starting point for overall health and well-being.

PATIENT SUCCESS STORIES

Sleep Disorders Center
Portable Home Sleep Study Report

Patient Name:					Patient ID:				
Date of Birth:					Chart Code:				
Weight:	125.0 lbs				Study Date:			10/17/23	
Height:	5' 3"				Age:			65	
BMI:	22.1				Sex:			Female	
Waist: 0"	Hip: 0"				Referring Physician:				

Comments: Moderate snoring
Total Recording Time (TRT) : 519.9 minutes

Respiratory and Snoring Events	Total#	Index	Duration (sec.)			Cardiac					
			Mean	Min.	Max.	Avg HR:	63.2	Min HR:	49.0	Max HR:	109.0
Central Apneas	0	0.0	0.0	0.0	0.0	Oximetry					
						Mean SpO2			94.2%		
Obstructive Apneas	0	0.0	0.0	0.0	0.0	Min SpO2			91.0%		
						Max SpO2			99.0%		
Mixed Apneas	0	0.0	0.0	0.0	0.0	SpO2 Range		%		Minutes	
Hypopneas	0	0.0	0.0	0.0	0.0	90-100 %		100.0%		517.4	
Apnea+Hypopnea	0	0.0	0.0	0.0	0.0	80-89 %		0.0%		0.0	
Snoring	0	0.0	0.0	0.0	0.0	70-79 %		0.0%		0.0	
Desaturations	0	0.0	0.0	0.0	0.0	60-69%		0.0%		0.0	
3% Hypopneas	0	0.0	0.0	0.0	0.0	50-59%		0.0%		0.0	
						< 50 %		0.0%		0.0	

Body Position	Snoring Volume Table dB(A)					Body Position	Supine	Prone	Left	Right	Non Supine
	Supine	Non-Supine	Right Side	Left Side	Prone	% Time in Pos	4.1%	0.5%	56.7%	37.4%	94.6%
Min	50.0	50.0	50.0	50.0	50.1	Snoring events	0	0	0	0	0
Max	72.5	74.0	74.0	64.2	53.6	Apnea+Hypopnea	0	0	0	0	0
Mean	59.0	57.6	57.7	57.3	-	Apnea-Hypopnea Index.	0.0	0.0	0.0	0.0	0.0

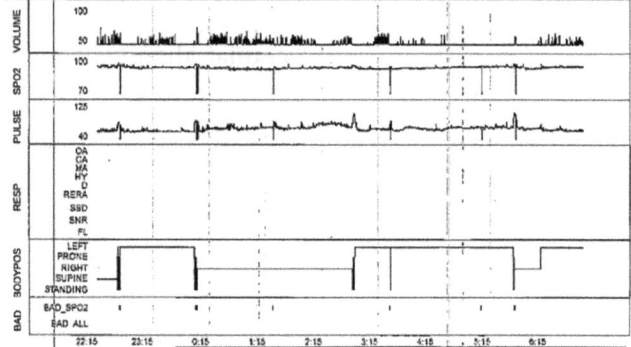

Patient	Apnea-Hypopnea Index	Severe	Moderate	Mild	Normal
	0.0	>30	15 to 30	5 to 15	<5

*Respiratory events are defined in the Assisted Scoring User Settings and in the User Guide. Final clinical decisions and degree of accuracy are the sole responsibility of the clinician using this software.
Powered by BRAEBON®

The sleep study above shows improved sleep apnea for Sarah after a year and a half of treatment.

CHAPTER 10

The Key to Successful Treatment

Embarking on a 12-to-18-month-long treatment requires, as it does with any other treatment, trust and an open and honest relationship between patient and healthcare provider. Unrealistic expectations of what is possible should be addressed before any treatment is started, and an attitude of gratitude on the part of the patient for receiving carefully designed treatment is paramount.

This book intends to guide you into understanding that there is a wider vision than just addressing teeth and bite. There is limited training with this modality, and it is up to the dentist, AFTER graduating from dental school, to pursue continued education from accredited sources to widen the narrow view of dental diagnostics and treatment.

Dental crime scenes of extractions and underdeveloped jaws are too common, leaving patients who trusted the professional handicapped with more problems than when they started. Outdated standards of care from years ago, when we didn't have the knowledge of how removing teeth instead of making space for them in the jaw was so detrimental, have left many patients with consequences like sleep apnea and TMD.

The job security is real: We extracted teeth when the patient was growing up because that was what we were taught to do, and now, as adults, these patients can't breathe due to underdeveloped jaws, so we treat them as sleep apnea patients. The dental student trusted what he/she was taught in the dental school and spent at least $500K in school tuition, only to be trained from a narrow-minded, tooth-only perspective. This has hurt the profession and patients alike.

There are no accredited TMD specialties in any dental school, only dentists who search for continuing education to help patients with pain and suffering when dysfunctional jaw joints produce symptoms.

Symptoms of dysautonomia relating to jaws and cervical spine misalignment need to be addressed comprehensively, not just in the dental chair but in a multispecialty full-body approach.

The gimmick treatment market, brought on by the advent of the professional patient who gets last-minute pseudo-clinical knowledge via Dr. Google, has undermined the trust between patient and dentist even more. We, as dentists, can't explain the whys of the problem in 5 to 10 minutes when understanding the problem, diagnosing it, and crafting a treatment plan requires knowledge acquired through years of investment into continued education and dedication to our work.

WHY THE LONG FACE?

Genetics, ethnicity, environment, or bad habits: what determines a dysfunctional face? Well, all of it! However, we should remember to focus on what we can actually control.

Dialing in the best practices for breathing and nutrition from birth will lead to proper growth and development into a healthy adult. Parents' vigilance on proper breathing, chewy natural foods, and non-toxic environments will optimize growth and development.

We can't unsee the problems once we recognize them, but how do we recognize them if there is not enough awareness brought in by preventive dental and medical information to our patient pool? And what if there is not enough dental education to train our young dentists?

I pointed out to a family member that the established open bite of their two-year-old baby was a problem stemming from improper, immature swallowing and bad tongue posture, only to be retorted with a "We are not worried about that. It will self-correct!" This reminds me of a saying I love:

> **When the patient is ready, the healer appears,**
> **and only then will proper treatment**
> **be accepted and implemented.**

The mental attachment to physiological dysfunction could create an identity. In this case, offering solutions to problems that the patient doesn't believe they have is futile, and even if they do recognize that there is a problem, there is often some type of connection to the dysfunction. The reasoning "Who would I be if I am all better?" or "This is the way I am; I don't need any fixing" will hinder any possibility of healing.

Lack of relational behavior and isolation while staring at our not-so-smart phones longer than physiologically acceptable with a hunched head forward posture has brought more cervical problems with repercussions in lower jaw positioning and temporomandibular joint health.

Over-the-counter solutions to these in the form of breathing workshops, sleep hygiene suggestions, and mini weekend courses that claim to address the root of all symptoms and problems abound. Some have mildly positive temporary results, but they all lack a proper professional diagnosis of the root of the problem and, as such, don't provide lasting relief. I can't teach proper breathing if there is no room for the tongue from lack of proper jaw development and inflamed nasal passages from constant mouth breathing. If the breathing apparatus is physiologically suboptimal, it needs to be addressed first.

We treat difficult patients who have tried many over-the-counter methods and some professional approaches but have not found relief. In my experience, the more complex the cranial pattern out of neutrality, the more difficult the patient, not just from a physiological point of view but also emotionally. They are tired of trying treatments and seeing no results, and understandably so.

The cranial vault holds our physiological abilities as well as our mental and emotional bodies. A compressed and torqued dura will have a negative effect on the nervous system. While emotional awareness and training can compensate for almost all deficiencies, getting to that point is not common. An emotional state of awareness that will compensate for a less-than-ideal physiology is reserved for a few.

Seeking neutrality in cranial patterns and posture and the possibility of proper breathing is the road to health and longevity at all levels. Bringing found conditions during the thorough evaluation to the patient's awareness and their acceptance and ownership of the presented findings is the first step on the road to health optimization and wellness.

CHAPTER 11

Challenges and Future of Dentistry

As with any new and innovative approach to healthcare, orthocranial dentistry faces a number of challenges and obstacles as it seeks to gain wider acceptance and adoption within the dental community. From limitations in insurance coverage to a lack of awareness and understanding among patients and providers, there are many factors that can hinder the growth and development of this promising field.

At the same time, the potential benefits of orthocranial dentistry are significant, offering a new paradigm for addressing the root causes of dental problems and promoting optimal health and wellness. As more research emerges and more patients and providers become aware of the transformative potential of this approach, it is likely that we will see continued growth and evolution in the years to come.

CHALLENGES IN ADOPTION AND ACCEPTANCE

One of the biggest challenges facing orthocranial dentistry is a lack of awareness and understanding among patients and providers. Because this approach differs from traditional orthodontics in significant ways, many individuals may be hesitant to explore it as an option for their dental care.

In addition, because orthocranial dentistry often requires significant time and financial investment, some patients may be deterred by the perceived costs and commitment involved. This can be particularly challenging for those without comprehensive dental insurance or with limited financial resources.

Another obstacle to widespread adoption is a lack of training and education among dental professionals. Because this approach requires specialized knowledge and skills, not all dentists are currently equipped to offer these services to their patients. This can limit access to care and make it difficult for patients to find qualified providers in their area.

OPPORTUNITIES FOR GROWTH AND ADVANCEMENT

Despite these challenges, the future of orthocranial dentistry is bright, with many exciting opportunities for growth and advancement in the years to come.

One key area of opportunity is in the realm of research and education. As more studies emerge documenting the efficacy and benefits, it is likely that more dental professionals will become interested in learning about and incorporating these techniques into their practices. This, in turn, can help increase access to care and raise awareness among patients about the potential benefits of this approach.

Another area of growth is in the development of new technologies and techniques to support treatment. For example, new software and 3D printing have brought in-house fabrication of dental devices with more accurate design and faster turnaround. Our 3D printers produce better-fitting custom appliances than ever before. Advanced imaging systems that allow data collection of bone and tissue structures are also part of 3D dentistry, allowing for more accurate fitting of different dental appliances.

Addressing pressing public health challenges, such as the rising prevalence of sleep apnea, temporomandibular joint disorders, and other chronic health conditions, by offering a wholistic, preventive approach to dental care, epigenetic, orthopedic, and orthocranial dentistry can help promote optimal health and wellness for individuals and communities alike.

Next Steps

As the field of orthopedic dentistry continues to grow and evolve, it is important for patients, providers, and policymakers alike to stay informed and engaged in the conversation. By advocating for increased access to care, supporting research and education, and raising awareness about the potential benefits of this approach, we can help ensure that more individuals have the opportunity to experience the transformative power of this type of wholistic dentistry.

I invite you to join me on this journey and become part of the growing movement toward orthocranial dentistry.

By working together and staying committed to the principles of epigenetic dentistry, we can help create a future in which everyone has access to the care and support they need to achieve optimal oral and overall health. So, let us embrace the challenges and opportunities that lie ahead and work toward a brighter, healthier future for all.

Conclusion

It's clear that the field of orthopedic dentistry represents a paradigm shift in the way we think about and deliver dental care. By focusing on the underlying causes of dental problems and taking a wholistic, patient-centered approach to treatment, orthocranial dentistry offers a promising new paradigm for promoting optimal oral and overall health. From addressing chronic pain and sleep disorders to promoting proper facial development and preventing common dental problems, the benefits of this approach are significant and far-reaching.

Throughout this book, we have explored the key principles and practices of epigenetic, orthopedic, and orthocranial dentistry, from the importance of proper diagnosis and treatment planning in promoting healthy facial development, alleviating pain, and improving breathing. We have also heard inspiring stories from patients whose lives have been transformed by this innovative approach and explored some of the challenges and opportunities facing the field as it continues to grow and evolve.

By embracing a wholistic, preventive approach and working collaboratively with other healthcare providers to address the unique needs of each patient's entire body—not just the teeth—we can help promote optimal health and wellness for individuals and communities alike.

At the same time, it is important to recognize that the journey toward widespread adoption and acceptance of orthocranial dentistry is ongoing and that there is still much work to be done to raise awareness, increase access to care, and support continued research and education in this field.

As a dentist and advocate for this type of approach in providing dental care, I am excited about the possibilities that lie ahead and remain committed to working towards a future in which everyone has access to the care and support they need and want to achieve optimal oral and overall health.

Whether you are a patient seeking a more wholistic approach to your dental care, a provider looking to expand your skillset and offer new services to your patients, or simply someone who is passionate about promoting optimal health and wellness, I invite you to join me on this journey and become a part of the growing movement toward health optimization and wellness.

Together, we can create a future in which dental care is not just about fixing teeth but about promoting optimal health and overall wellness for all. So, let us embrace the challenges and opportunities that lie ahead and work toward a brighter, healthier future for ourselves and the generations to come.

I hope that this book has inspired you to think differently about your oral health and to explore the transformative potential of this innovative approach. Remember, your mouth is the gateway to your overall health and wellness, and by taking a wholistic, proactive approach to your dental care, you can unlock the key to a lifetime of optimal vitality and well-being.

If you feel that any of this information has sparked your interest and you can relate to any of the symptoms and stories described in this book, please call to set up an in-depth evaluation:

212-765-1877

or email info@drlauratorrado.com

About the Author

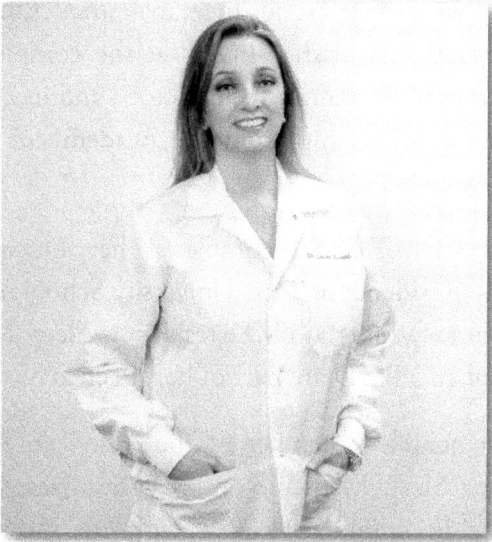

Dr Laura Torrado has been designing functional smiles since 1989. A graduate from NYC College of Dentistry and a previous degree in dentistry from Uruguay defines a career where learning never ends

She has continued her studies in full mouth rehabilitation and fixed and removable prosthetics at NYU.

ABOUT THE AUTHOR

At Buffalo State University ,she completed the advance program in esthetic dentistry and is an avid participant in numerous continuing education courses both nationally and internationally

Dr. Torrado is a Pankey scholar and a graduate of the Kois Dental Center in Seattle whose curriculum includes 9 courses with the latest advances in aesthetics, implants, and restorative dentistry. In 2004, she completed her certification in Invisalign Technologies, and in 2005, she received her fellowship from the Academy of General Dentistry.

In 2015, Dr Torrado completed her Dental Sleep Medicine Residency at Tufts University School of Dental Medicine as well as a TMD residency. Sleep Medicine and facial and TMD are part of her practice .

She is a qualified member of the American Academy of Dental Sleep Medicine and also completed a mini residency in craniofacial pain with the Academy of Cranio Facial Pain.

She is a member of the International College of Cranio-Mandibular Orthopedics, the American Dental Association and the Academy of General Dentistry.